Marvel's "Marvelous" Yoga

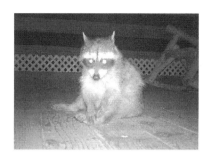

Marvel's "Marvelous" Yoga
Yoga for People, Inspired by a Raccoon

Andrea Rumery

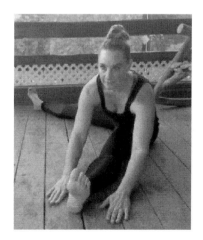

Marvel's "Marvelous" Yoga

DEDICATION

I dedicate this book to my loyal and amusing husband, Mark Rumery. He humorously took these photos of me and I love him for always telling me that he loves me, to make my dreams come true, and to enjoy myself; my friend, Kitty Cantrell, who generously provided the idea for this book and shared the copyrighted photos of Marvel the raccoon; and of course to Marvel herself.

ACKNOWLEDGMENTS

Thank you to my aunt, Pamala Redhawk, for the astonishing and inspiring cover art. My deep appreciation also goes to Lois Niven for designing and meticulously editing this book and to Yvonne Hunsaker for encouraging me to keep writing. I also want to acknowledge my yoga teacher, Joy Bennett, for sharing her passion for yoga and teaching me how to teach yoga.

      I am thankful to all who find the value in this marvelous little book. My happiness and recognition obviously reaches out to Marvel the raccoon and all animals that teach us so much about the world around us. Animal poses are significant in yoga. May we remember that we can co-exist and are all one. I believe that it is important to live in harmony with nature, each other, and our highest purpose. Namaste.

      In yoga, sequencing is important as well as preparatory poses, precautions, contraindications, and learning the benefits of each pose. In this book, the poses start with warm ups and each pose prepares the yoga student for the next pose. I found, after analyzing the raccoon's behavior, they naturally move in ways that support healthy reproduction, good digestion, and detoxification. How marvelous is that?

Andrea Rumery, LMT, RYT

FOREWORD

I have known "Marvel" the raccoon since she was a baby, when her mother and siblings used to play on my back porch every night. Marvel has been here for over 4 years now, and has brought me much joy and laughter, watching her nightly antics.

Different people drift in and out of our lives, but the special ones become lifelong friends. Marvel has allowed me to be a part of her life and has taught me much about what it means to be a free independent person. I have watched her raise her children, seen her gentleness with them, and also her strength and determination defending them from dangers. Life is hard on a wild animal, but Marvel continues to live it "her way", the best she can.

My back porch is marvels "special place". She comes to relax, enjoy a treat of fresh grapes I leave out for her, and just enjoy herself. I have a trail camera set up on the porch, so I can see some of what she does without disturbing her. After she has had her treat of grapes, she likes to have a nap, or stretch, or roll around. Some of the positions she gets into resemble "yoga" moves.

The first time I met Andrea, I was at a musical gathering of friends. There were drums, didgeridoos, and other instruments being played around a crackling fire. Andrea began to dance. She is a yoga teacher and her flexibility makes for some enchanting dancing. Andrea seems to always be smiling. You can't be around her and not feel energized by her presence.

It seemed only natural that Andrea and Marvel should combine their talents for bringing happiness with this book. I hope you enjoy them as much as I do!

Kitty Cantrell
Ramona, CA
2019

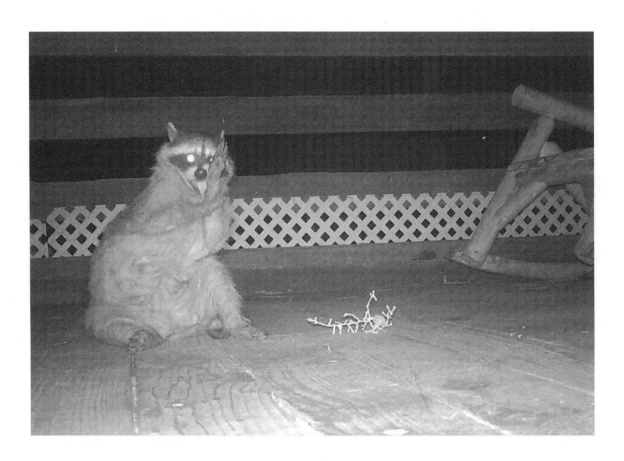

Garudasana

This pose increases flexibility in the wrists, shoulders, and between the shoulder blades. This asana increases confidence.

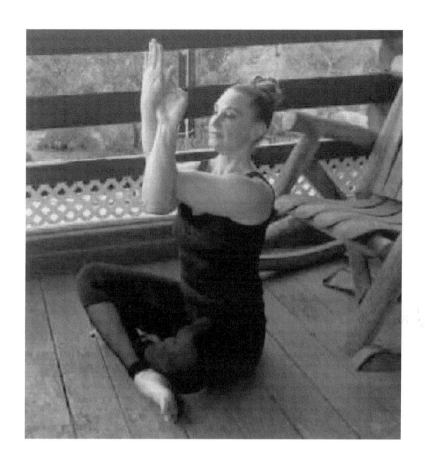

Eagle Arms

Proceed cautiously if you have low blood pressure or a shoulder injury.

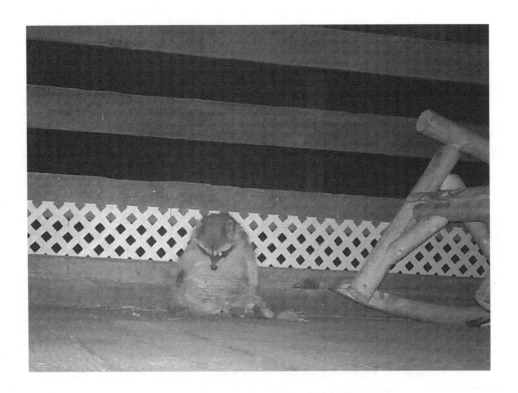

Chin to Chest

On an exhale, softly drop your chin toward your chest. Look inside your heart as you stretch and relax the back of your neck. On the inhale lift your chest and look up at the ceiling without forcing it. Exhale to neutral.

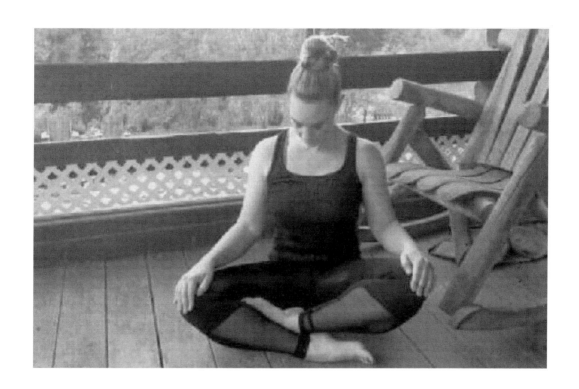

Chin to Chest

Follow with neck twists and rotations. Be slow and gentle.

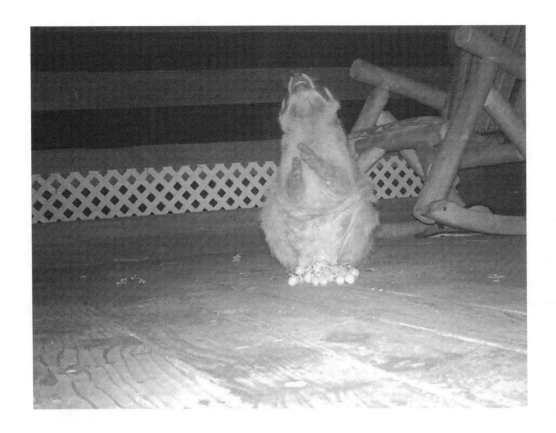

Laughing Yoga

When Marvel the raccoon eats the grapes, she throws her head back so the juice runs down her throat, not wasting a drop. What a lesson! Drink in all of life's sweetness. Grapes have their own healing properties such as helping to lower the risk of blood clots.

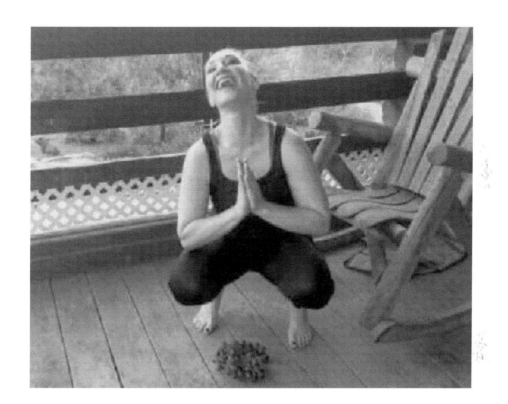

Laughing Yoga

Laughing yoga can increase immunity, digestive and bowel health, bone strength, and memory. Laughing maintains blood pressure, regulates menstruation, and relieves headache. It may also decrease pain, and help in cancer prevention.

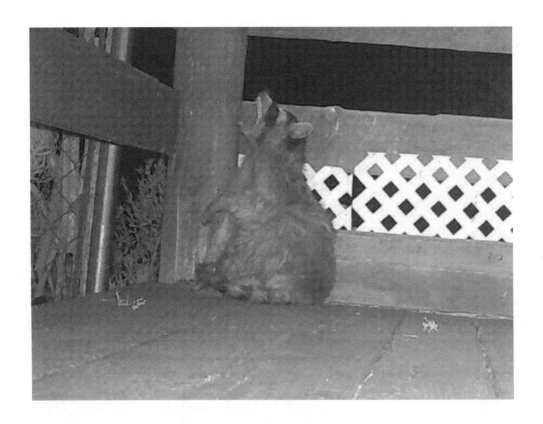

Look Up and Open Jaw

As you inhale, lift your chest slightly to protect your neck and look up to the sky. Exhale. On your next inhale, release your bottom jaw and open your mouth to soften and relax the jaw. Take a soothing breath or two and on the exhale, close your jaw loosely and bring your head back to neutral.

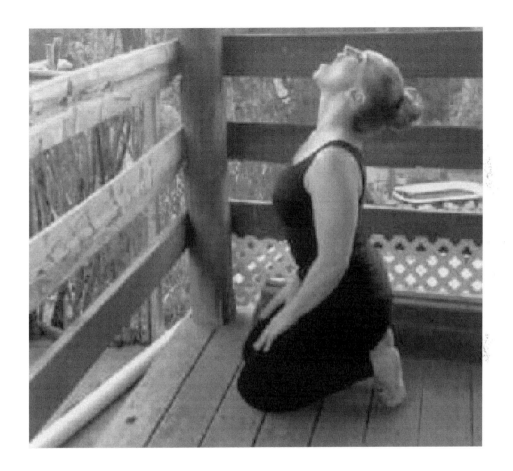

Look Up and Open Jaw

This pose is to release pelvic tension, chronic tension in the jaw joint, and to reduce headache pain.

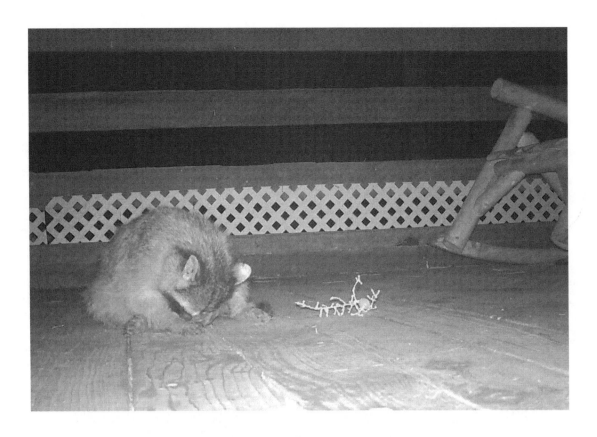

Baddha Konasana

This is a great preparatory pose for Boat Pose (Paripurna Navasana).
This pose improves posture, stretches inner thighs, and relieves sciatic pain.

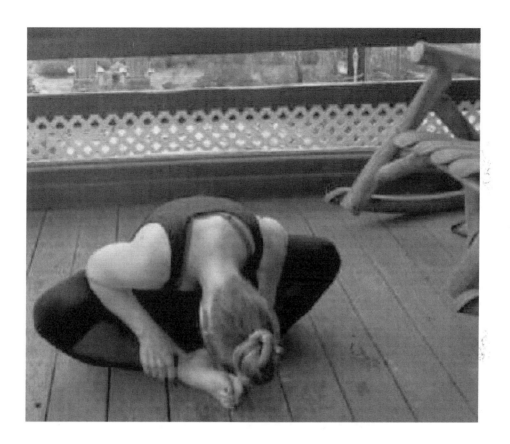

Bound Angle Pose

It helps with menstrual cramps and menopause symptoms. It is also stimulates the bladder, kidneys, ovaries, prostate gland, and abdominal organs.

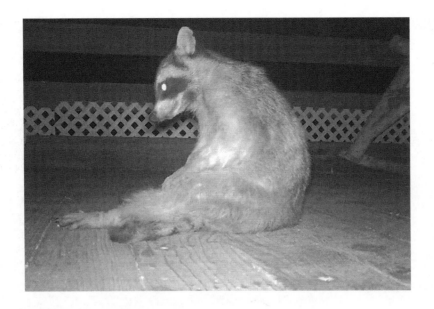

Paschimottanasana

This pose can be tricky, especially for beginners. If you're particularly tight, you can use a folded blanket under your seat and rolled ones under your knees. The goal is not to see how far your forehead can get to your knees. It's about lowering your stress levels and finding calmness in the stretch. Some will find that their spine is so full of tension that stretching the hamstrings are a secondary reason for the stretch.

It is helpful to inhale the breath into the tight regions then exhale out the old energy. It may be challenging to bring the breath in deep the further down you get but that is where all the benefits are. It is important to hinge at the waist with an elongated spine on the exhale to allow the hips to become more flexible.

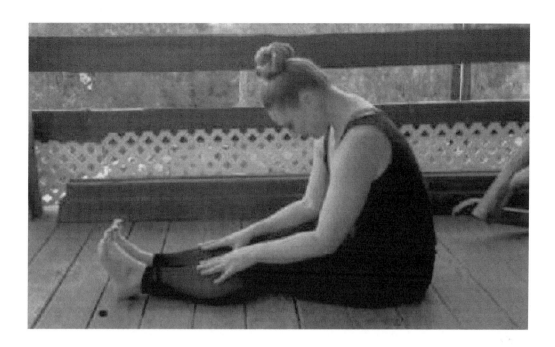

Seated Forward Fold

Once you have warmed up in this pose with several breaths, on your exhale, you may wish to drop your chin carefully to your chest and let your spine become limp, or bring your forehead towards your knees. Benefits include increased digestion, female reproduction health, and lowering headache pain and high blood pressure. It's also wonderful for the kidneys and liver.

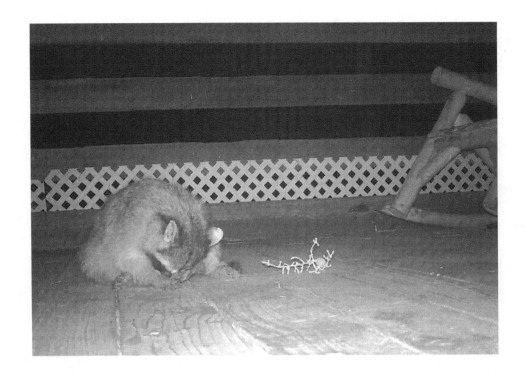

Upavistha

Use caution if you have a low back injury and you may wish to sit on a folded blanket for more comfort. Keep in mind to go only as far as you comfortably can using props to help you relax deeper. Inhale and sit tall through your spine. On your exhale, hinge at the waist and without arching the back or hunching over, lower your torso toward the earth. Rest your head and relax your neck and the end of your stretch. Keep the spine lengthened the whole time. Flex the feet and engage the thigh muscles to keep the legs straight. When your third eye reaches the earth or a prop, enjoy the intense ability to reach deeper wisdom and cleansing of the third eye.

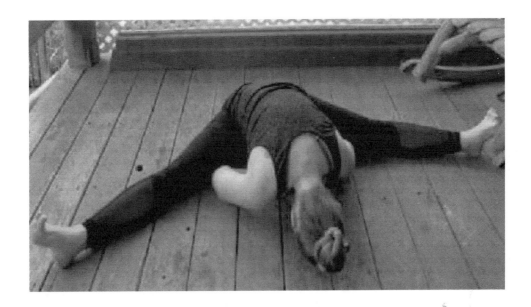

Seated Wide Legged Forward Fold

Breathe into the tight areas and exhale the tension stored there. This pose is wonderful for colon health, to detox the kidneys, relieve arthritis, and can relieve sciatic issues.

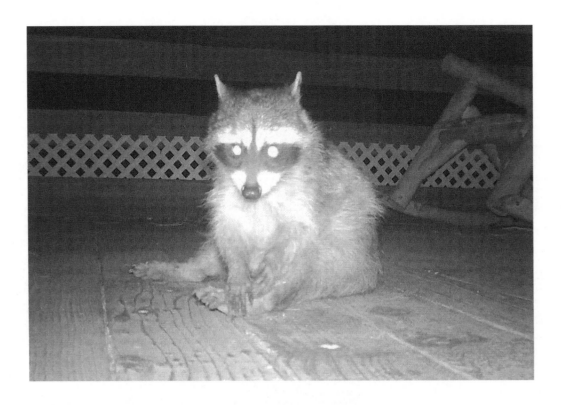

Upavistha Konasana

This variation strengthens the spinal cord and the core while stimulating the abdominal organs. Be cautious if you have a low back injury by using a folded blanket under your seat. It's a great way to detox your kidney and ease arthritis. It may help relieve sciatic nerve pain.

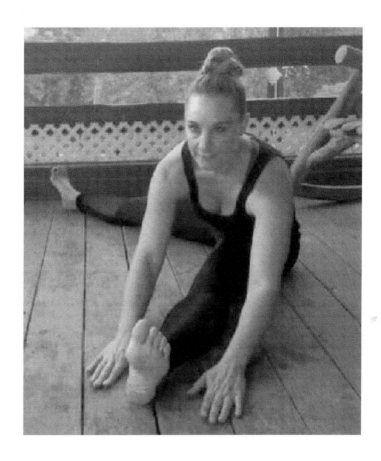

Seated Wide Legged Angled Fold

Inhale, lengthen the spine and sit tall and grounded. On the exhale twist your upper body so that your belly button faces your knee. On your next exhale, hinge at the waist being careful not to round the back or neck and flex your body aiming for forehead to knee placement. Deep and elongated breaths are key. Twist to the other side.

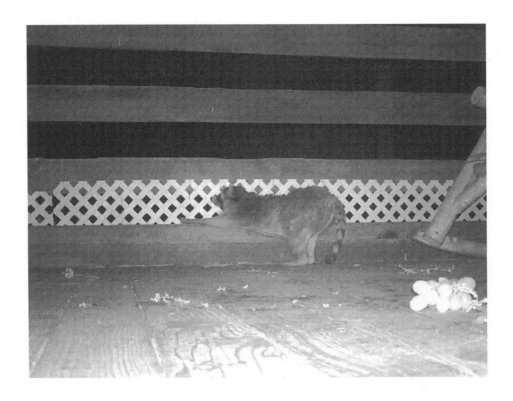

Adho Mukha Svanasana

This is a variation, instead of the hands being on the Earth, you can have them on the wall. Stand facing the wall with your hands on the wall about shoulder height. Inhale and push your into hands and elongate your spine, exhale and begin to walk your hands down or walk your feet away to feel a stretch in the spine and hamstrings. You might not go as far down as the pictures show. To lift out, do so with an inhale.

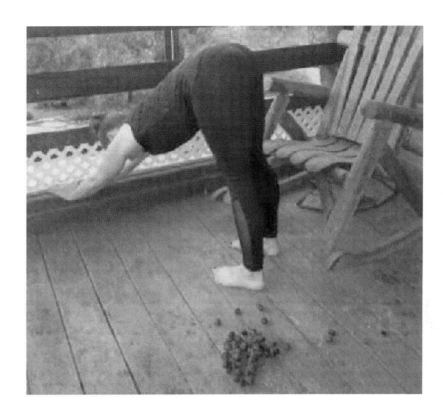

Downward facing Raccoon

This pose is excellent for osteoporosis prevention, increases digestion, relieves headaches, lower back and sciatic pain, lower blood pressure and asthmatic symptoms, and soothes the nervous system which in turn relieves stress and depression. Use with caution if you are late term pregnant, have diarrhea, carpal tunnel, or high blood pressure. Don't forget your grapes!

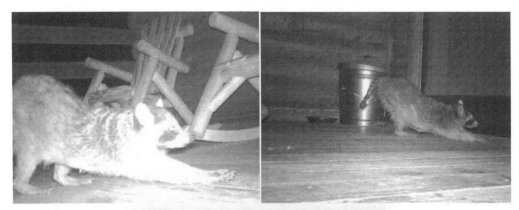

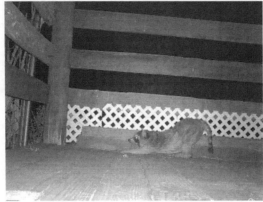

Uttana Shishosana

Extend your hands and arms out keeping strength in them as you exhale your seat only half way toward the heels. It's kind of like a cross between Child's Pose and Down Dog.

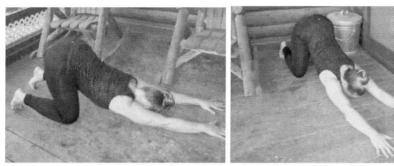

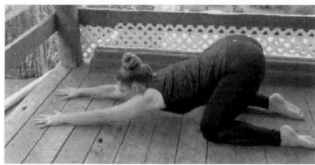

Extended Puppy Pose

Use caution if you have a knee, shoulder, back, or arm injury. This pose will calm your mind, decrease insomnia, diminish chronic stress, headache, and is just overall soothing. It stretches the spine and curling your toes will give them a nice stretch.

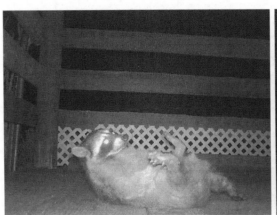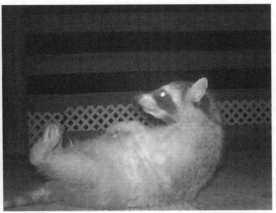

Paripurna Navasana

This is a great pose to strengthen your core muscles and hip flexors, improve balance and digestion, and to stimulate intestines, prostate gland, thyroid, and kidneys. It will also relieve stress. Practice reaching your seat into the Earth and ground while elongating your entire spine to the Heavens. All the while, press out through your heels and reach through the hands. Use your core to stabilize and breathe in wisdom.

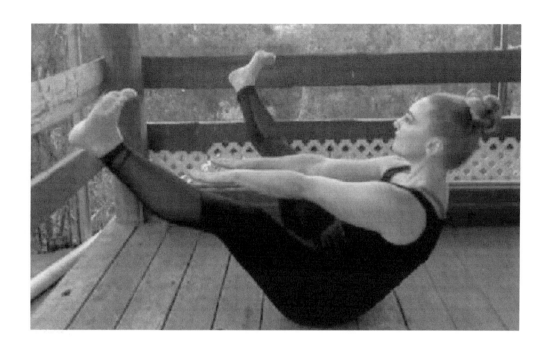

Boat Pose

Contraindications to this pose include asthma, headache, insomnia, pregnancy, low blood pressure, menstruation, and diarrhea. Use caution if you have a neck injury.

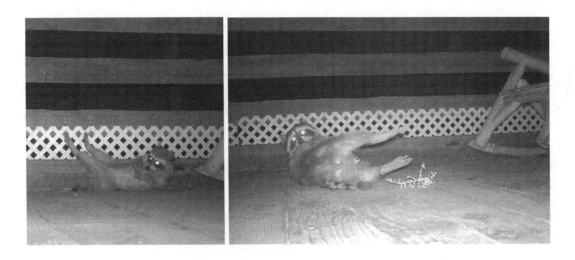

Paripurna Navasana

This pose can reduce back pain and stress while increasing spinal flexion. It aids in detoxing and improves digestion. Inhale, reach and extend all of yourself, exhale to twist to the side. Inhale to center and exhale to the opposite side.

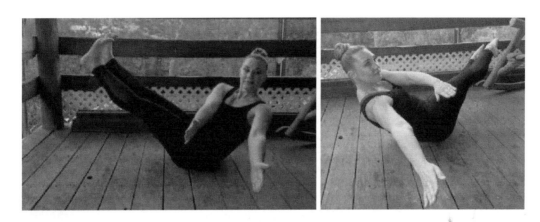

Boat Pose with a Twist

Do as many as you can as long as you can maintain good posture. Feel the difference in the abdominal muscles when you point your toes compared to flexing the feet.

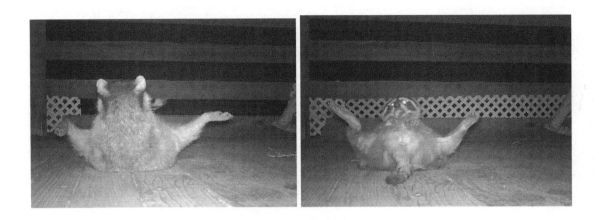

Paripurna Navasana

This is Boat Pose again and leave it to Marvel to teach us that it is okay to stick out your tongue out and have fun. In yoga we call this the Goddess tongue. It helps us to release anxiety, ego, and fear.

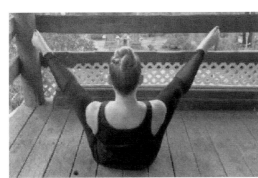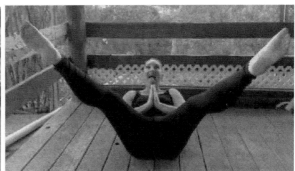

Boat Pose

It feels good to stick your tongue out. Try it! It will stretch your jaw muscles and joints and release tension in our throat. Pay special attention to keeping your spine lengthened and legs strong and straight. Breathe fully.

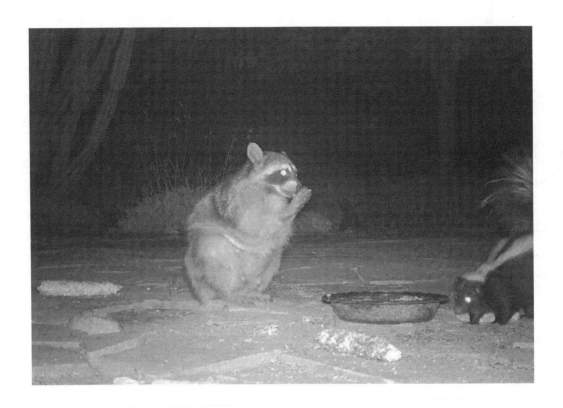

Malasana Squat with Anjali Mudra

This pose strengthens the entire lower body. Squatting increases sexual energy and brings blood flow to the pelvis. It stretches the calves, thighs, low back, and whole torso.

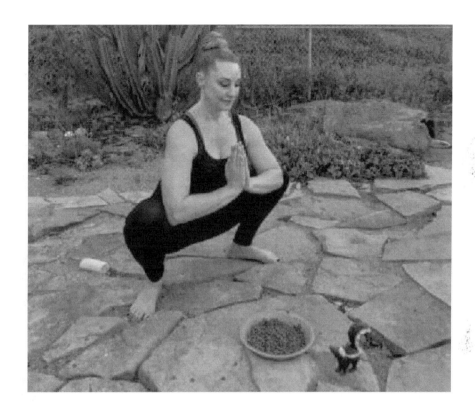

Prayer Hands ~ Namaste

Namaste is a Sanskrit word for "bowing to". Offer, with prayer hands, a salutation to the timeless and universal energy within you and outside of you. This unifies your left and right brain, nourishes your body, mind, and soul, and centers you. Namaste also means that you notice and honor the Divine spark in others.

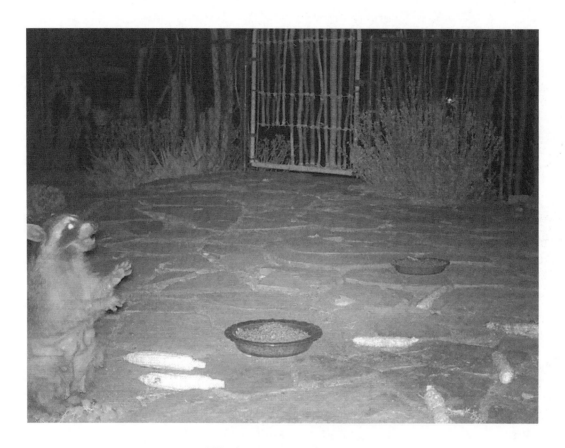

Vajrasana Pose

Kneeling on the Earth with toes curled under stretches the toes releases the fascia in the feet, and strengthens the arches. It also improves posture, but use caution if you have knee sensitivity.

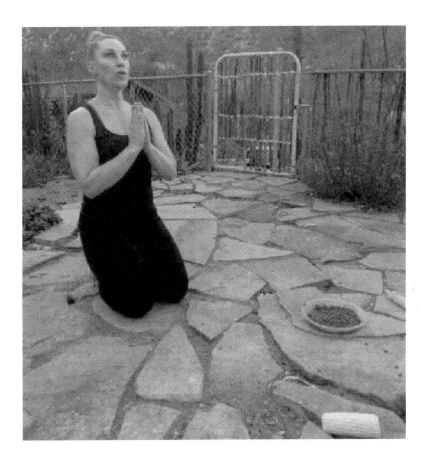

Thunderbolt with Om (Aum)

Om is the primordial sound that is chanted, aloud or silently, that signifies the essence of the Infinite Consciousness, encompassing all sounds. It represents the deep sleep, dream, and waking states. Focusing on this mantra will reduce mental distractions.

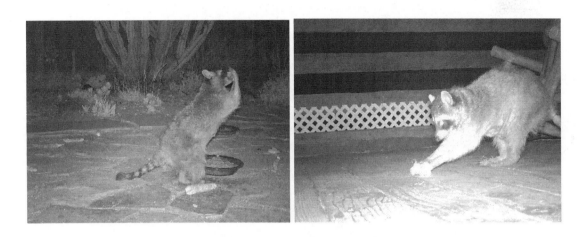

Upavistha Konasana

Stand facing East. Inhale reach up and place your hands in prayer position. In this modified version, exhale and hinge at the waist into a forward fold. Inhale and roll up slowly one vertebrae at a time lifting the head last.

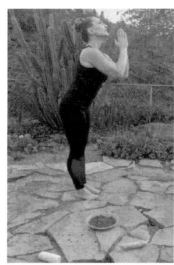 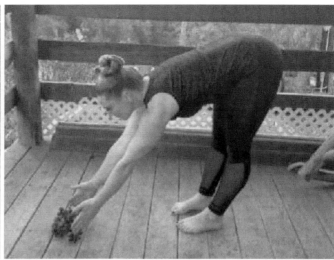

Sun Salutations

I like to do sun salutations also to the South, West, and North. Sun Salutations bring in much needed Prana (intelligent vital life force and breath), improve blood circulation and purification, and strengthen your body.

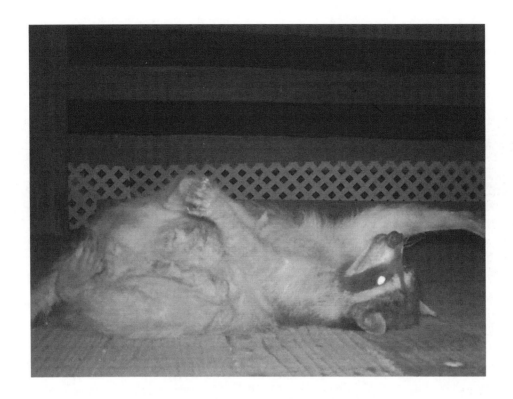

Supta Padangusthasana

This raccoon is so naturally wise! This pose heightens focus, relieves sciatic, low back, and menstrual pain. It helps regulate blood pressure, aids in fertility and digestion, tones the arches of the feet, stretches the hamstrings, calves, hips, and arms. Contraindications include diarrhea, uncontrolled high blood pressure, and headache. The twisted variation of this pose stretches the IT band and low back.

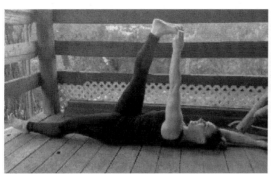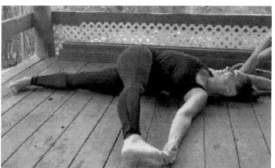

Reclining Hand to Big Toe

This is a pranic (energy strengthening) and yang (masculine) pose.
Everything is strong and aligned. Keep your muscles tight against the bone,
limbs lengthened, and breath deep and rhythmic like a deep ocean. Use
exhales to contract the muscles and inhales to extend them.

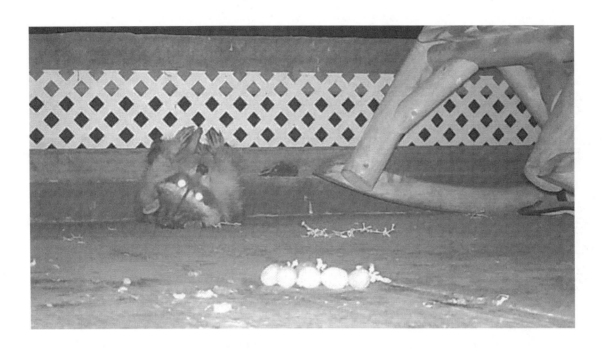

Ananda Balasana

Be careful if you have a knee injury otherwise, hold your feet and aim your knees toward your armpits. Rock side to side massaging your spine and it's not complete until you put that happy baby smile on your face. Smiling lowers your heart rate and blood pressure. It promotes health and a good mood. This is one happy raccoon!

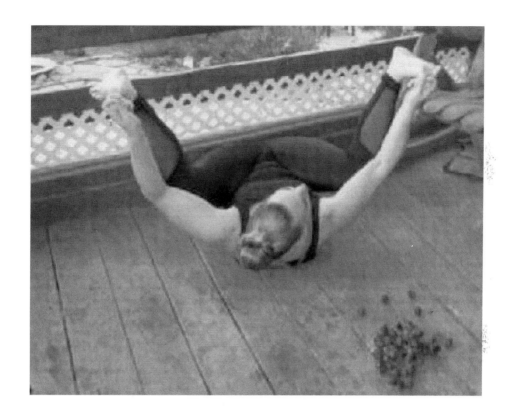

Happy Baby

Happy Baby Pose lengthens the spine and muscles between the shoulder blades. When your mind is in overdrive and your brain needs a break, practice this. This pose can help prevent leg injuries, especially to the groin and hamstrings. There is even a slight chest opening here which soothes our heart chakra.

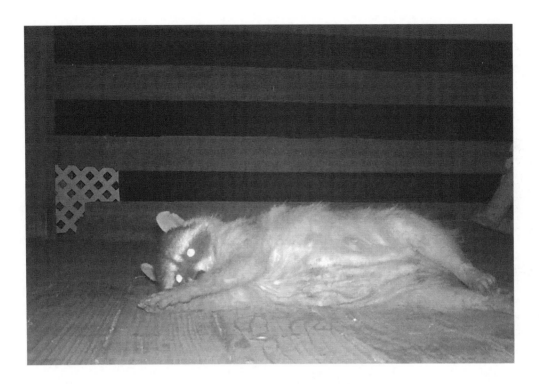

Parsava Savasana

Savasana is a relaxation pose generally used at the end of a yoga practice and there are no muscles, mantras, pranayama (breath exercise), or intentions used. It's just a time for you to just be. Try not to fall asleep or think about the past or things to be done after class. It helps to visually guide yourself to a beautiful meadow, mountain, or ocean beach to relax before Savasana.

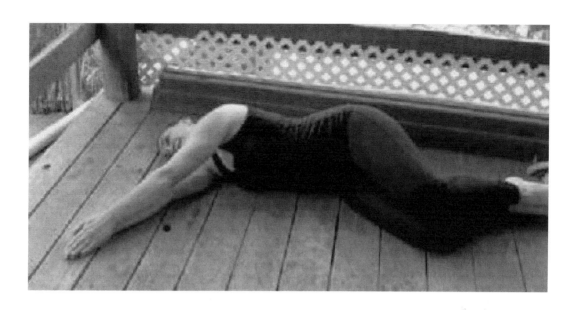

Side Lying Stacked Hands

Lying on the right is so revitalizing with added benefits of slowing the nervous system and activates the left nostril and the Ida Nadi (energy channel) for increased blood flow. On this side, the internal organs won't suppress the heart function and impede the blood circulation. Enjoy this pose for at least five minutes.

~ NAMASTE ~

About The Author

Andrea is Nationally Certified as a massage therapist and is a member of Yoga Alliance. She has been teaching yoga for nearly three years providing peaceful, loving, and fun classes for a yoga studio as well as a fitness center in her nature-filled community. Her educational background in massage therapy and energy work for over 20 years has given Andrea a solid foundation for assisting her students in reaching deep inner peace and healing. "Give yourself permission to feel good" is her motto.